THE BUSY BODY

by
Penny Ingham
and
Colin Shelbourn

SUMMERSDALE

Summersdale Publishers Ltd
46 West Street
Chichester
West Sussex
PO19 1RP
UK

www.summersdale.com

Printed and bound in Denmark.
Nørhaven Paperback A/S, Viborg

ISBN 1 84024 225 6

To Polly and Russell,
for giving me direction (PI)

To Mary, onward and upward (CS)

CONTENTS

INTRODUCTION   **6**
how to use this book – chapter sections explained
– read this now

1 ANYONE FOR TENSION?   **15**
observing tension – starting to break those habits
– recognising what you are doing to yourself

2 FIRST STOP AND THINK   **22**
introducing the idea of a thinking space – pause to reorganise –
the power of thought

3 IS WORK A PAIN IN THE NECK?   **27**
head balancing for beginners – the relationship of head, neck and
back – how to become taller, feel better and look more confident

4 RECHARGING THE BATTERIES   **36**
why you should lie down three times a day – flat out benefits for
the spine – practising vital body maintenance

5 ARE YOU SITTING COMFORTABLY?   **49**
sitting can damage your health – find your sit bones
– balance in the chair – sitting: a whole body thing

6 CHAIRMANSHIP   **63**
become master of the chair – desk and table manners without
strain – an easier, freer way of performing activities whilst sitting

7 REACH FOR THE STAPLER   **76**
simple actions cause problems – damage limitation
– learn to lean longer

8 EYE CAN SEE CLEARLY NOW   **84**

the eyes have it – the way you look at the world affects your well-being – have a visual spritzer – the holiday effect

9 GETTING ABOUT   **90**

standing and walking tall – first steps to freer and lighter movement

10 THE WORLD ON YOUR SHOULDERS   **107**

allow those shoulders to drop – re-educate your arms – smile across the shoulders

11 FLEXIBLE FRIENDS   **120**

exploring all the parts – regain lost mobility – where have your moving parts been today?

12 LIFT OFF   **129**

bend those knees – climb those stairs – be buoyant

13 DON'T HOLD YOUR BREATH   **144**

breathing more usefully – let go the out breath – whisper an 'ahh' and relax

14 WHERE NEXT?   **151**

you never stop – signposts for the future – where to find a guide

APPENDIX 1 – BODY MAP   **153**

a guide to the body

APPENDIX 2 – THE POSTURE POST-ITS   **157**

essential affirmations

INTRODUCTION

How are you holding this book? Is your chin jutting out? Head pulled back? Shoulders hunched? If you are standing, is all the weight on one leg? How are your hips? Hitched to one side? Is your lower back tight?

If you are sitting, are you arching your back or slumping in the chair? And by the way, how is your breathing?

Do you suffer from backache, tiredness, stiffness in the joints, digestive problems, lack of energy, shortness of breath, onset of RSI (Repetitive Strain Injury), irritability, or low self-esteem?

If so, you need *The Busy Body*.

The way that we habitually stand, sit and move can cause all the symptoms above. Few of us have the alert, easy posture we had as children. Over the years we have acquired damaging postural habits which incorporate and reinforce the strain and tension of everyday living. But because we have learnt these habits, we can unlearn them.

Once you understand the problems poor posture can cause, you can use that understanding as the key to getting back in control of your busy life.

Furthermore, the principles in *The Busy Body* can be incorporated into every day of your life. All the time you are at work you can be using the techniques in this book to make yourself feel better, fresher, more in control and more energised.

The Busy Body sets out a programme for change. It is a body owner's handbook for you to regain and maintain ease, poise and pain-free posture.

HOW TO USE THIS BOOK

Each chapter can be used as a self-contained piece of work but your understanding will build up chapter by chapter and a glance through the whole book will prepare you for more detailed work.

Chapters 1 to 4 form the foundation of the book and are fundamental to understanding later chapters. Begin with these and then you are ready to dip into any of the remaining chapters out of sequence to follow the exercises.

Appendix 1 – Body Map – is also essential if you want to successfully navigate round your body.

Each chapter contains five sections: The Problem, The Exercises, The Principle, The Posture Post-it and Reorganise Your Life.

THE PROBLEM

An unwelcome symptom such as backache is your body giving you useful feedback. Listen to it. The aches, pains and stiffness may well be the result of something you are doing to yourself. Over the years, you may have acquired damaging postural habits or methods of working and moving which put unnecessary strain on your body. But, if you are doing harm to yourself, you can learn to undo it. What you need is this book and a little insight, patience and perseverance.

It is important to realise that body problems are interrelated. That stiffness in your fingers, for example, may be caused by the way you sit or are getting in and out of your chair. The symptoms listed in this section are a rough indicator of what might be going wrong; all the chapters in the book will be beneficial, even if you think you need to address only one particular problem.

THE EXERCISES

These are quite unlike conventional keep-fit exercises. They are habit-breakers. They require mental rather than physical effort. They are designed to examine and remedy the tense and over-effortful way in which you have been making everyday actions, and to encourage your body to revert to its natural, tension-free way of doing things. Take your time over each exercise – if you do it too quickly, your muscles will take over and repeat the old, habitual way of doing things.

We use words and images which help you make less effort. For example we say *let* your elbows drop to your sides, *allow* your shoulders to widen, *think of* a string taking the crown of your head upwards. All these phrases help you to naturally adopt these ideas, which is the very opposite of forcing the body into a good posture.

When you attempt the exercises, do so with a friendly and interested attitude. The quality of your attention is a key factor in the effectiveness of each exercise. If you perform them quickly in a let's-get-this-done sort of way, your body will miss the point. Staying with the process can be difficult at first. If you find that your mind is elsewhere, find another time when you are in a more receptive mood. Work on these exercises when you feel you can give them your full attention and then you will be making real changes.

Remember that just as you acquired damaging postural habits by repeating the same thing over and over again, so you need to unlearn the habits by repeating the exercises. Like skilled craftsmen or musicians you never stop practising. Continue to work on yourself.

THE PRINCIPLE

In this section we explain more about why and how you might have acquired a particular problem and the relevance of the exercises. It puts the work you are doing into a useful context. You will find it helpful to read these sections along with a glance at the Body Map.

THE POSTURE POST-IT

The chapter in a nutshell – thoughts you repeat to yourself to direct your body into its easier, natural posture. They act as antidotes to bad postural habits and reinforce the new you.

They work in a similar way to affirmations. They help to change the unhelpful script most of us have running around our heads most of the time (for example substituting the positive 'I can do this' for the negative 'I can't do that'). Repetition is the key factor to affirmations; the positive thought consciously replaces the negative until a new way of thinking is formed.

Thoughts work on our body in a similar, very potent way. The Post-its help remind you of useful thoughts on posture. We offer some suggestions for these but feel free to add your own – making up your own will help you think about the work you are doing on yourself. But keep them positive – 'do' is more useful than 'don't' and is less likely to introduce the wrong idea. For instance, if we say: 'Don't think of an elephant!', what is the first thing you think of? Exactly.

Once you have your thoughts, distribute them about your desk, computer screen, anywhere you will see and be reminded of them.

REORGANISE YOUR LIFE

Practical tips and hints on how to modify your lifestyle and environment to help maintain the new you. Be a rugged individualist; look after yourself in a practical, organised way and get back in control of your body.

... AND FINALLY

The Busy Body is aimed at working on yourself in the workplace but not exclusively so. If it is really not feasible to do a particular exercise in your everyday environment, try it as soon as you get home. (You will, in any case, want to continue the process at home and out of normal work hours.) Although you can treat the exercises individually, the effect of the book is cumulative. Any of the exercises will be a useful re-education of your body, performed wherever, whenever you can. The more you do, the more you get out of it. It's not just about work, it's not just about home – it's about life.

CHAPTER 1
ANYONE FOR TENSION?

THE PROBLEM
Are you doing too much?

Most of us are tense to a degree – you might be breathless, have a bad back, headache, digestion problems or just feel more tired than you think you should be. You're doing too much.

It's nothing to do with a heartless boss or unsympathetic co-workers, it's you! You can be lying on the beach and still be doing too much. It's all down to the habits you've learned since you were a child.

THE EXERCISES
Exercise 1:

To begin with, here's a really easy demonstration of muscle tension and how to release it. (This is also a good exercise in observation.)

Hold your hand (either one will do) in front of you at face level, palm side-on, forearm vertical. Your wrist needs to be visible for this exercise.

Keeping your hand open, tighten your wrist muscles. You will feel a pull towards your elbow. Notice that this measurably shortens the distance between the tips of your fingers and your elbow, and arches your hand.

Tense   *Released*

Now release the muscle tension. Your hand is still supported in an upright position, but you are doing much less work and the distance between your fingertips and elbow is much longer. You've released tension to allow your hand and forearm to lengthen upwards.

This is a precise analogy of everything postural we will learn during the course of this book.

Exercise 2:
Sitting at a table with a cup in front of you, place one hand on your bicep and with your other hand, pick up the cup. How much effort do you need?

If you feel muscles pulling from the elbow to the shoulder, you are doing too much. You have a nice little muscle in your forearm which is more than adequate for the task. Try it again, minimising the effort all the time. Hinge, don't heave.

PRINCIPLE

Tension – what is it and why do our muscles grow tense?

We become tense at work for a whole variety of reasons which can be categorised into two groups – psychological and physical (mechanical).

Some psychological factors would include: not enough personal space on the tube, not enough office space, the urge to leave the meeting NOW and not being able to, the primitive urge to have a punch-up with someone at the meeting when politeness and promotion prospects prohibit us.

Physical factors would include: chairs sloping the wrong way (see Chapter 5), unsatisfactory work stations, cramped working conditions and so on.

When tense, the posture we adopt is the startle response. That is, whatever the stimulus, we respond in the same way: we tighten our necks, pull our heads back and shorten the whole length of our spines. We have entered 'flight or fight' mode. We make these unnecessary and damaging movements whenever we make an action – however minor. We've learnt the habit – through repetition in formative years – of gearing ourselves up, ready for action, instead of going smoothly into that action.

When we're psycho-logically tense, our muscles are tense. One way to help cope with the psychological pres-sure is to begin to deal with the muscular ten-sion. For example, unclench that jaw. If your jaw is tight, the rest of your body can-not be relaxed – other muscles will tighten as well; it is a cumulative effect.

REORGANISE YOUR LIFE

Give yourself time to observe these energy-wasting habits. Do a personal tension audit: when you make a move, perform an action or respond to a request, stop, relax, observe what you're about to do and break the habit of tension.

When you're busy at work, it is easy to forget about your body unless it becomes stiff or painful. But you don't have to ignore your body awareness in order to concentrate on something else. To begin with, you may need to take time out to observe what you are doing. As you become more practised, you will be more aware of how you are moving, sitting or standing whilst engaged in everyday activities. It is a skill which can be learned – a slightly different mode of thinking with continuing benefits.

CHAPTER 2
FIRST STOP AND THINK

THE PROBLEM

You want to stop being tense but you don't know how. People tell you to relax but no matter how you try, somehow it eludes you. So how do you do it?

THE EXERCISES

Exercise 1:

You can do this sitting or standing. Cross your arms. Now cross them the other way. Not so easy is it? Notice how much you had to reorganise your approach and think through the movement before crossing your arms in the unaccustomed way.

Make a point of trying a few actions with your non-dominant side, for example: which arm goes into the jacket first? Same hand on the computer mouse? Telephone always on the same side? Trousers on with the same leg first? You have to think it through to reorganise these activities to favour your non-dominant side. This will make you more sensitive to body balance.

Exercise 2:
For this you need a small, unbreakable object such as a ball of paper or a plastic cup. Standing or sitting, prepare to throw the object from one hand to the other. Extend the catching hand out in front of you. Usually you would move this hand to catch the object but in this exercise you choose not to – you let it remain still.

With your throwing hand, throw the object into your catching hand without moving the latter. The object may fall but never mind. If it lands in your hand, clasp it, but if it misses, let it go. Under no circumstances are you to move your catching hand to intercept the object. The purpose of this exercise is to test your ability to resist the impulse to move.

Try this a few times with both your dominant and non-dominant hand doing the throwing. As with the previous exercise you will find you have to engage your brain to actively inhibit the catching reflex.

THE PRINCIPLE

Stopping and thinking are twin activities which should be complementary.

Stopping – putting a pause in between resolving to make an action and then performing it – allows for thinking time. You can then act in the newly organised, unfamiliar way. You will be giving yourself more options and be more in control. This means that you are potentially more in control of your tension and the internal factors contributing to it.

As you work your way through this book, you will find that you are being encouraged to pause (inhibit your reflexes), think about what you are about to do and direct your body to go about the action in the new way (sometimes using images as a tool to help you).

In this way, you will find that you do not have to be a slave to damaging postural habits. You can learn to observe, think about what you are doing and reorganise the way you are about to do it.

By making your mind work harder, your body will have an easier time.

REORGANISE YOUR LIFE

Begin by organising the filing cabinet inside your head. Dispose of outdated notions of posture. Posture which requires strenuous effort (chin out, chest up) can go straight in the bin. Instead, start working with the idea that to achieve poise, balance and elegance of movement, you can do less work by thinking in a new way about your

25

body. The exercises, thoughtfully performed, will help you recognise when you are making too much effort.

Thinking organises your body to do less, not more.

CHAPTER 3
IS WORK A PAIN IN THE NECK?

THE PROBLEM

Do you suffer from a stiff neck or tension headaches – for example, when sitting at a desk or keyboard?

You're probably tensing your neck and pulling your head back, without realising it. If your neck is tight, your chin juts forward and you're compressing your spine. You're probably so used to this posture that it feels completely normal. Sitting up straight is the usual reaction but this is not a good way to go about it and is more effort; you need to attend to the way you balance your head on your neck.

THE EXERCISES

Exercise 1:

Begin by sitting on an office chair or dining chair (not your favourite armchair). Imagine a string attached to the crown of your head and going up to the ceiling. (The crown is not the top of your head – it is farther back.)

A friendly puppeteer is about to pull on the string, to draw you gently upwards, crown first. As the puppeteer pulls, your neck begins to lengthen. This will make you aware of the muscles at the back of your neck. Think of these muscles relaxing.

As the neck muscles release and lengthen, the back of your neck can't help but move towards the back of your collar. As your crown is drawn upwards, your chin drops and your forehead rolls slightly forward and up.

By imagining a puppeteer doing the work, you are not stiffening or forcing your neck into a new position but allowing it to happen naturally. The less you tighten the back of your neck, the longer it becomes; muscles contract as you tighten them and lengthen when they relax.

As your neck muscles relax and lengthen, your head, neck and back realign themselves and you regain your natural poise.

Exercise 2:

Find a hand mirror and a larger mirror. Turn your back on the large mirror and align the hand mirror to view the reflection of the back of your neck in the large mirror.

Now think through the images in Exercise 1.

Notice that if you don't stiffen your neck but allow it to release upwards, it will ease back into your collar, your head will roll very slightly forward (as if rather more weight has dropped into your forehead) and, as your neck muscles continue to release tension, you will see that you have rather more back of neck. You will find that the more you think of releasing those neck muscles, rather than tightening them in a 'sit up straight' manner, the longer your neck and spine become. This is a very useful look and learn exercise.

THE PRINCIPLE

Your head weighs around five kilograms. We're so used to this weight that we don't notice it. Next time you're in the supermarket, pick up five kilogram bags of sugar; that's what your neck has to carry every day.

Your head is carried on the top of your spine. It balances at the *atlanto-occipital* joint, the uppermost joint of your spine, deep inside your head. This joint is perhaps higher in the skull than you imagined.

The front of your head is heavier than the back. When your head is perfectly balanced, this extra weight rolls your forehead slightly forward at the pivot, the *atlanto-occipital* joint.

In everyday life, most of us tend to carry our heads poorly balanced: chin forward, neck compressed, taking the world on the chin. In so doing, we're making far too much effort to carry our heads. Long term, this is damaging.

There are two layers of muscles involved in the head, neck and back. One layer is the external, moving musculature, the other is the internal, postural musculature. We don't need to tighten the moving muscles to balance our heads when we're in our normal, upright position (sitting or standing).

It's worth reminding ourselves that when our muscles release, they lengthen. If your neck muscles are released, you cannot help but be taller. By allowing the crown of your head to release up, your head rolls slightly forward and your neck – which was tightened – begins to ease back and straighten. With the pressure off, your neck and the full extent of your spine lengthen and realign. Balancing your head becomes effortless. You are more relaxed, taller, you look leaner and you are feeling better already.

REORGANISE YOUR LIFE

If you work at a computer screen, it's important to get the screen in the correct position. This has been written about many times before but now you've got a new factor to take into account.

Once you've lengthened your neck, your forehead has rolled slightly forwards and your eye level is no longer where it was. In fact, it may feel very unfamiliar – as though you are peering out from under your eyelashes. Expect this to take time to become familiar.

If your screen was previously correctly positioned (and that's a big if) you'll now find it needs to be lowered.

Before you start heaving the screen about, try it with a book. Hold it at arm's length where your screen is now, focus on a word or phrase, then lower the book as you lengthen your neck. Feel where the book is most comfortable to read. That's where your screen should be.

By the way, this does not mean that you must hold your head vertical at all times. With released neck muscles and a balanced head, it is easy to move your head naturally when required. (Practise now for Chapter 8!)

CHAPTER 4
RECHARGING THE BATTERIES

THE PROBLEM
Fatigued, lack of stamina, bone tired, the Monday morning feeling which lasts all week?

You probably won't realise it unless your back is giving you pain, but those feelings of fatigue are most likely coming from your spine.

Apart from sleeping at night, how many times do you lie down in any 24 hour period? What everyone's spine needs is a 20 minute period of lying down, ideally twice during the working day – once around lunch time and again 5 hours later.

THE EXERCISE
You will need a clear floor space which is warm and comfortable to lie on. You also need a small stack of paperback books or magazines to support your head and, ideally, 20 minutes (although even 5 minutes is beneficial). Not all workplaces have a clear floor space but you can usually find

somewhere (a meeting room, the chairman's office). Don't be self-conscious – it is important to do this around the middle of the day.

Lie down on your back, with your head resting on the stack of books and your knees pointing towards the ceiling.

Your head should be supported by the books with your neck clear. The contact point with the books is the lower, flatter part of the back of your head, just below the bump of the *occiput*. (The bony protuberance at the back of the head – see Appendix 1.)

Adjust the height of the stack to establish head, neck and back alignment; with too few books, your chin will stick up towards the ceiling, with too many your chin will press down into your throat. The books should support your head in such a way that your chin tilts slightly towards your chest with a gentle slope from forehead to chin.

A good rule of thumb is that the back of your neck is approximately parallel to the floor; you can check this by running three or four fingers between your neck and the floor, making a note of the height of the stack for next time.

Let your elbows rest on the floor as far out to the side as possible, with your hands palms down, resting on your body. Relax your wrists and feel the full weight of your hands on your body – take your time over this and feel the tension dropping out of your wrists.

Place your feet on the floor as near to your bottom as feels comfortable, without strain, with the inside of your feet in line with the outside of your hips.

Your knees point to the ceiling. Relax your leg muscles so your kneecaps are over your little toes; if you are too tense, your knees will pull together and the kneecaps will be over your big toes. This is quite a subtle point but a good indicator of how relaxed your leg muscles have become. As with the wrists, spend time working on this.

When your knees are at a point of balance, you may feel them trembling slightly. This is usual – as you practise, you'll achieve the right point without the trembling. You are learning quite a sophisticated balancing act.

Relax your ankles and bring your attention to the underside of your feet; if your legs are appropriately balanced, the weight will distribute around the outside of your feet – a perfect footprint – and not down on the arch. Now you can begin!

To bring yourself into the present moment and closer to your sensations – listen.

Absorb the sounds around you as though you are collecting them. Some will be sounds from the room around you, some from outside and some will be the sounds of your own body, such as your breathing.

Now think of your spine releasing tension and lengthening and widening. Feel the support of the floor beneath you and think of sinking into soft sand, your body imprint getting longer and wider. As you lose tension, you make more contact with the surface beneath you.

The exercise so far is going to be beneficial to your back. However, to take it further we can extend the exercise and realise even more benefits:

Picture a line connecting two joints of your body; for example, your right knee and left shoulder. Imagine that line becoming longer as your muscles release.

Now switch your attention to your right wrist and left shoulder. Again, picture the line connecting them becoming longer.

Work around your whole body in this manner, not forgetting the many joints in your feet and hands and the 24 joints of your spine, extending up into your skull. It does not matter too much

which joints you choose – they can be next to each other or on opposite sides of the body – the benefit is the same.

As you can see, if any colleagues ask what you are doing, you are perfectly justified in telling them: 'working!'

THE PRINCIPLE

The discs of your spine perform the vital function of insulating your vertebrae from physical trauma (the everyday impact of moving around). The discs are like sponges, absorbing spinal fluid to act as highly efficient shock absorbers.

7 a.m.   noon

After five hours of being upright, they need recharging to maintain their resilience. Without this recharging, after a further five hours the discs will have compressed even further, lost fluid and be well below optimum condition. They will now be much less resilient than when you got out of bed in the morning. This is one reason why most people lose measurable height during the course of a day.

without lying down ————————

result of lying in semi-supine --------

During a typical working day, what do we do? Most of us spend hours at a desk, sitting in meetings or in a vehicle or otherwise remaining upright. So long as we stay vertical, the essential process of disc recharging cannot happen.

Lie down in the semi-supine position described above and three things happen:

At a mechanical level, the discs absorb the fluid they need and are once more able to perform their important task – along with the vertebrae – of forming a protective tunnel for the spinal cord, from which nerves run linking every part of your body to your brain.

Secondly, by lying in the semi-supine position and using the floor as a reference, you can feel where your back is over-arched.

Your spine is naturally gently curved for strength and resilience – so gently that your back should feel flat on the floor when your knees are raised.

The more the underside of your body contacts the floor, the less tense you are. Tension would have you arching away from the floor. The books help you realign your head, neck and back.

Turn this book through 90 degrees to show the lying figure upright, and you will see how your back should look whilst you are sitting (see Chapter 5).

Finally, when you get up again, having realigned your head, neck and back, lengthened and widened your body and having recharged the discs of your spine, you will be feeling much clearer, more relaxed and focused. And, incidentally, you will be taller! The combination of plumped up discs and muscle lengthening can restore your height by as much as three centimetres. Your discs recharge as you work on releasing tension from your muscles. You are effectively working and relaxing at the same time.

As you learn to release muscle tension, you will remain taller during the course of the day and so have less height to regain during the lying down work. The mechanical advantages of lying down are still vital to the well-being of your spine and so to the well-being of you. Remember that your discs still need regular rehydrating.

REORGANISE YOUR LIFE

Think of this as a challenge. It may be difficult to arrange but most workplaces have floor space where you can lie down. Rather than have a coffee break, have a lying down break – the benefits will be far greater.

Having understood the principles and experienced the effects, you will feel confident enough to make this lying down work an essential part of your life. Make a point of putting it in your diary or organiser. You will be valuing yourself, improving your personal performance and your colleagues will respond positively to that.

You will also gain benefits if you can schedule a brief session of lying down work before tackling something stressful or demanding – for example, before an important meeting – especially if it has been a long time since your last session. You will feel clearer and more capable before tackling the challenge.

Be brave. Let your well-being infiltrate the workplace.

CHAPTER 5
ARE YOU SITTING COMFORTABLY?

THE PROBLEM
Most of us sit badly. Problems associated with poor sitting include fatigue, lower back problems, sciatic pain, poor breathing, bad digestion, poor circulation and lumber disc problems.

All these problems can be caused by faulty posture whilst sitting. Sitting puts three times the strain on your spine as ordinary standing (and we shouldn't stand for long, either … but see Chapter 9).

THE EXERCISES
Exercise 1:
Most of us don't know how to sit and it takes practice. You might find that sitting in a poised, balanced and less stressful way seems so unfamiliar – and uses your back muscles in such a different way – that it feels uncomfortable at first.

Find a chair with as firm a seat as possible – note that it's what you sit on that's important, not the chair back. The seat should be horizontal or, ideally, slightly sloping downwards from back to front (never the other way round).

When sitting, your legs should be at right angles to your body or, ideally, your hips higher than your knees. Your feet should be comfortably apart, fully supported by the floor.

Sitting on the chair, first find your sit bones by turning your hands palms up and sitting on them. Feel the sharper sit bones towards the back of the base of your bottom.

Now you remove your hands. Let the weight of your torso be fully and equally supported down through your sit bones – think of them as little feet in your bottom.

Slide a hand down the length of your spine until the palm rests on the *sacrum* and your middle finger on the *coccyx*, or tailbone. (See Appendix I – Body Map.) Allow the whole of this area to drop by releasing the muscles. Your buttocks will release outwards, like an inverted fan opening. You will begin to feel your sit bones contacting the chair more fully. This will seem unfamiliar if you associate good sitting with the classroom technique of tightening muscles to sit bolt upright.

You can actually feel the tension dropping out of your back as your tailbone drops. If your back feels slumped, it is because you are forgetting to allow your neck to lengthen and your head to roll forward and upwards. The release of muscle tension and alignment of your head, neck and back are crucial and indispensable parts of sitting comfortably.

Think of both your neck and tailbone lengthening out of your spine.

Although you may associate the relaxing of your lower back with slumping, the important difference is in the buoyancy of your head as it balances on the top of your   lengthening spine.

Exercise 2:

Put one hand on the front of your body, just under your breastbone. Allow yourself to push your chin forward and pull your head back to go into the old, bad way of sitting. Feel how this pushes that area of your gut down. Is it any wonder we get stomach problems through bad posture?

Now try this: put both hands on your sides, spanning the distance between the bottom of your ribs and the top of your pelvis.

The more space there is there, the better. And if you find one side has less space than the other, then this reflects an asymmetrical sitting position. To correct this, think of your head and spine as a plumb line passing down through your body and that you are sitting equally on both sit bones.

Exercise 3:

Now redirect your attention to your legs and feet. When you're sitting, your other important area of support is the floor. If your legs are balanced and supported, your knees will slightly drift out from the centre line. Think of your knees in relation to your toes. In good sitting, your kneecaps should be over your little toes, not over your big toes.

Try tightening your legs together – as though clutching a champagne bottle between your knees – then release them and you'll notice that your knees naturally drift away from each other.

You may find that you need to relax your ankles to let the soles of your feet remain in full contact with the floor.

Now with your torso supported by the chair, your feet supported by the floor and your head balanced, you really are sitting comfortably.

THE PRINCIPLE

Sitting is a whole body thing. Your head and pelvis balance each other and they can do it wrongly:

Even in poised sitting there is three times more strain on your spine than when standing. All around your joints there are feedback mechanisms which cause your muscles to tighten when you are off-balance. If you stop fighting gravity and regain your balance, you will be using them less and making much less effort.

Your sit bones, formed from the lower part of your pelvis, are two rockers which make it possible to balance the weight of your torso in sitting. Sitting balanced, the weight of your head is distributed along the whole length of your spine. When we sit badly, that weight falls directly onto the lumber region.

This is a major cause of slipped disc conditions and why they nearly always happen in this part of the spine. You do just as much harm sitting in a self-consciously tense, upright position as sitting in a slumped collapse.

This is neither slumped nor strained – it's poised.
 Once you get used to the feel of being balanced when you sit, you'll stay relaxed, comfortable and happier for longer.

REORGANISE YOUR LIFE

Make sure your chair height is correct – your lower legs should be vertical and your thighs either horizontal or sloping slightly downwards from hips to knees.

If your chair is badly designed, modify it! Invest in a specialist wedge-shaped cushion (or have one made from a block of hard foam) to raise your hips slightly higher than your knees. You may also need to modify the height of your desk.

If your chair's upholstery is very soft – or if your chair seat slopes back – sit on the front edge to support your sit bones. (If your chair is on castors, be very careful how you do this – invest in some carpet protectors to stop your chair sliding backwards.)

Make the surface of your chair support you – if it is too soft, make a hard cushion from a piece of plywood covered in soft fabric.

It is important to remember that the floor and your chair are there to support you. If you don't accept their support, you will be tense.

'It might not be very elegant but think how much better I'll look when I'm sitting on it.'

CHAPTER 6
CHAIRMANSHIP

THE PROBLEM
In the previous chapter, we looked at postural problems whilst sitting in a chair. Those problems (principally of the lower back) are exacerbated when you become active: leaning forward to type, write, read or when getting up and sitting down. The effect is cumulative.

Building on the work in the last chapter, now is the time to take it further and become master of the chair!

THE EXERCISES
Exercise 1:
You can either do this sitting at a desk or table, or by imagining that there is one in front of you. This exercise should take you at least five minutes – do not rush it.

We are going to practise the movement you have to make to go forward from sitting position to, for example, eat, write or work at a desk. For simplicity, leave your hands resting palms up on your lap – at the moment your head, spine and lower body are enough to be thinking about.

Sit on a chair with as firm a seat as possible. Your legs should be at right angles to your body – or, ideally, hips higher than knees – sit bones in contact with the seat of the chair, feet flat on the floor, knees and ankles relaxed, head nicely poised on top of your spine.

Locate your hips. This is important – they are almost certainly not where you think they are. These are not the part of you that holds your trousers up – that's the brim of your pelvis. Your hips are much further down, the bony protuberances at the very top of your legs on the outside, and deep in the groin on the inside.

PELVIS

HIPS

ELVIS

Your hips are the hinges which allow your seated body to go forward to the desk or table. You will be pivoting slowly at your hips; your torso and spine working as one unit.

Now you're ready to begin moving. Work on this exercise very slowly, pausing to organise yourself. The aim is to remain relaxed, aligned, lengthened and poised throughout.

Think of your forehead being magnetised towards the work area of your desk in front of you. You are being drawn forward but with your head, neck and back moving as one. This image will start the momentum and allow your torso to drift gently forwards.

PIVOT

As you go forwards, free your neck and back of tension. We want to maintain the length and freedom we achieved in Chapter 3.

Think of your neck continuing to lengthen and your lower spine – your tailbone – continuing to drop, until you arrive at a position for comfortable working.

Your relaxed legs continue to do nothing, except remain balanced. If your legs tighten, loosen those knees.

The return journey reverses this process; the movement is initiated by dropping slightly more weight into your tailbone and heels, the counterbalancing effect causing you to rock gently back into the upright sitting position, once more pivoting at your hips.

The movement does not start by pulling your head back, otherwise you will scrunch the back of your neck and arch the small of your back.

Throughout both parts of the exercise, be careful to notice and avoid any tendency to swerve your torso, head or knees to the right or left.

This exercise retrains your body to move much more easily and naturally.

Exercise 2:

Standing up from sitting couldn't be simpler but, of course, it could be simpler than we make it.

Sit on the chair as before. Be particularly conscious of the balance of your head on your neck, the chair supporting your torso and the floor under your feet. Think of the undersides of your feet. Although you will be using the whole underside (except the arches) to bear your weight as you stand, most of the weight – around 60 per cent – will be in your heels.

Now move nearer to the edge of your seat and bring your feet back until your heels fall in a line just behind your knees.

Think through the activity ahead. From sitting to standing requires that you remain balanced all the time and that you go through the process of standing up by leaving one supporting object (the chair) in favour of giving all your weight to the other (the floor).

Think of your forehead being magnetised forwards. Rocking on your sit bones, allow your torso to drift gently forwards until it is sufficiently over your heels for you to straighten your legs easily into the standing position.

You'll know by now that a common mistake is to start the movement by tightening your neck, pulling back the head and thrusting the chin forward, as though coming up for air. Check that this isn't happening as it can be extraordinarily difficult to resist. Without this tension, you feel light and buoyant as your head leads you forward and upwards.

Keep dropping your tailbone as you stand, with your weight predominantly in your heels.

Sitting down into the chair reverses the process! Think of it as a kind of interrupted squat – the chair being the interruption.

As soon as your bottom reaches the chair seat, let yourself be fully supported again by the chair and the floor. Now you are sitting comfortably again.

Exercise 3:
Try standing up with your eyes shut. You will be much more aware of keeping your balance as you move, a key factor in good posture.

Take note of how you moved. Using these observations, try standing again with your eyes open, incorporating the more secure, and therefore balanced way you moved when you had your eyes shut.

THE PRINCIPLE
Sitting is not passive. Most of us have developed a range of bad habits associated with sitting, or getting in and out of a chair. The primary bad habit is beginning an action by pulling the head back and tightening the neck.

Having established a balanced sitting posture (as in Chapter 5), learning to move forward in a comfortable, balanced manner provides a foundation for a whole range of further activities.

Unless we're conscious of the way in which we do this, leaning forward falls into the classic stimulus-response pattern; our work is there in front of us and we react by reaching towards it without thinking about how we are getting there. Result – we are using far more effort than we need to for something which is a simple, repetitive and everyday part of our lives.

With the sit bones fully supported by the chair, and your feet supported by the floor, we are perfectly balanced. We don't need to spring into action by getting chin, legs, arms and shoulders involved, simply to lean forward.

Sitting is as much to do with the head as the bottom – remember that the head weighs around five kilograms. Leaning forward is a matter of adjusting your weight slightly and letting gravity do the work. Throughout, we allow the spine to work as one unit, carrying the head and body forward without undue effort.

When we get into a chair in a thoughtless and disorganised way, using our back instead of our legs, we stay like that and so retain bad posture.

When we get out of the chair in an unbalanced and disorganised way, we are using our spines when we should be using our legs to carry our weight up into standing position.

The job of standing and sitting down should be done by the legs, not the spine, which should remain at ease throughout.

POSTURE POST IT
pivot
at the
hips

REORGANISE YOUR LIFE

To help you feel secure when getting in and out of a chair, make sure it is not going to move when you sit down – restrict those castors. Most importantly of all, don't sit in it too long. Visit the water-cooler more often!

If you work at a computer, most machines have an alarm which can be set to chime gently every half hour, reminding you to get up and move around. You will be astonished at how easy it is to let two chimes slip by in quick succession without getting up. Failing that, invest in a egg timer – think free-range and move!

CHAPTER 7
REACH FOR THE STAPLER

THE PROBLEM

Middle and low back ache? Pain and stiffness in arms and shoulders?

When we reach and stretch from a sitting position, we can inadvertently put a tremendous strain on our middle and lower back, particularly if the movement is repeated during the course of the day. This, of course, is common when we are sitting at a desk, reaching for the phone, that urgent memo or the coffee cup on the far side of the keyboard.

This is a classic example of how a simple action can cause damage because we do it repeatedly, without thought.

THE EXERCISE

This may seem a very simple, everyday thing to do but follow the exercise slowly and gently and you will see an immediate benefit.

From a sitting position, you are going to be reaching for something just out of reach on your right. Your body will continue to face forwards.

Find a suitable office chair so you can sit and feel the contact of the seat with your sit bones. Your feet should be flat on the floor, the chair and floor fully supporting you (as in Chapter 5).

Your hands drop down by your sides, arms and shoulders relaxed, string taking head and neck upwards so your spine is lengthening.

Letting your eyes lead, gently turn your head to the right to look for the object you want to pick up.

Extend your right arm towards the object, an imaginary string leading your fingers towards it. Your shoulder remains relaxed and down – the more your muscles release and your shoulder drops, the longer your reach becomes. Most people simply do not believe this until they have tried it.

Once you feel that your arm has extended to its fullest amount, then, and only then, begin to gently lean into the movement.

Now, check where those sit bones are. They should both still be in contact with the chair. The likelihood is that the area around your left sit bone has begun to tighten and rise.

Think of relaxing and dropping this area as you gently lean towards your object.

Both sit bones keep contact with the chair and you are relaxing the sides of your torso. Your reach increases. You are increasing the length between your right fingertips and your left sit bone.

Think of the arm movement coming from the whole of your back and not just from your shoulder. You pay out the movement like a measuring tape extending from a reel.

To return to the upright position, think of increasing the length of your RIGHT side, so that you rock back into the vertical position.

Important: do not pull on your left side and be careful not to let your dominant knee go in towards the centre line as you return to the upright.

Repeat these movements, reaching to your left.

THE PRINCIPLE

When we reach for something it is easy to tense up and go for it. This is entirely counterproductive. By stopping and thinking, you enjoy the full, released length of your arms and your body remains relaxed, energised and your muscles retain their full suppleness and length.

Rock climbers understand this better than most. When balanced on a tiny foothold and stretching towards a handhold which seems at first to be out of reach, relaxing the shoulder allows the climber to gain the hold. Tightening up the shoulder, arm and hand would have the effect of shortening the climber's reach.

REORGANISE YOUR LIFE

The obvious point of reorganisation is to put things within easy reach. But don't overdo this – put a few lightweight, regularly used items just out of reach as an excuse to try out the exercises above and let yourself enjoy the new feeling of being longer and leaner.

Finally, if you have to reach for something behind you, make sure that the whole of your body goes round with you. Do not try and twist the upper half of your body by tensing your knees and legs and corkscrewing your spine.

CHAPTER 8
EYE CAN SEE CLEARLY NOW

THE PROBLEM
Stiff neck, fatigue, boredom, lack of energy, lethargy, rainy days and Mondays get you down all week?

THE EXERCISES
Exercise 1:
Stand and find an inanimate object at around eye level to focus on. Keeping focused on this object all the time, start moving your head around very slowly and in all sorts of movements, while keeping your feet where they are. For example, you might explore leaning your head backwards so that you are looking down the length of your nose as you drop back, bending your knees to stay balanced.

Or try turning as far as possible to the left, keeping your eyes on your chosen object.

Explore the number of movements you can make whilst maintaining eye contact with the object.

Exercise 2:

The previous exercise encourages your eyes to move. Now that your eyes are limbered up, try this:

Sit and imagine that you are about to park your car in a space behind you. Try miming this and notice how far your head goes round before you have to reach to undo the seat belt.

Now sit and look straight ahead. This time, let your eyes go all the way round before your head starts to move. Think of your eyes towing your head around. You will find that your head goes round much further than before.

As your head reaches its new finishing point, allow the rest of your torso to spiral after it in a lengthening movement from the sit bones and hips (which, if they are moving freely, means that you will be loose in your knee joints).

Now return – with your eyes leading – back to your original position.

Go through this again to the other side.

Exercise 3:

Give yourself a visual spritzer.

The next time you walk into your workplace – or any place or situation that you feel is boringly familiar – talk yourself into focusing on the objects around you. See the sharpness of the edges, the colours, the shadows and shapes. Give everything around you the sort of attention you might give if you were seeing it for the first time.

Exercise 4:

Another visual spritzer.

When sitting at your desk, focus on a point at eye level in front of you and allow yourself to become aware of your peripheral vision. Without moving your head or eyes, how much can you see to either side of you?

Whilst remaining focused on the point in front of you, think of lengthening your neck, allowing your head to roll forward and up and become aware of how much farther your peripheral vision extends behind you.

THE PRINCIPLE

When we are in negative states – under pressure and anxious or under-stretched and bored, or worse still, both of these situations at the same time – we develop unhelpful and debilitating ways of dealing with them; we employ what might be called the 'don't ask' look, deliberately avoiding eye contact with others. We look through our surroundings rather than at them.

These are our ways of dealing with situations we don't like, but the sad fact is that these are futile tactics – they just don't work. Not only that, they actually under-stimulate your nervous system; if your eyes are open, they need to be alert and focused. If your eyes are not focused, you will feel progressively more tired and tense as they day goes on because part of you is not functioning as it should. And remember that focused eyes look more attractive.

One of the reasons holidays and excursions are so beneficial is that the novelty of that bit of scenery or that picture at an exhibition invites your eyes to focus and to stay focused. This very damaging habit of not focusing is what we are addressing in Exercise 3.

Your eyes also become very tired when fixed for long periods of time on, for example, a computer screen. All these exercises will help you address that problem, as they invite you to unfix your gaze and vary your focal length.

Related to this is another lost art, that of our eyes leading – as in Exercise 2. If you ask a child to look at a bird directly above, that child's eyes will travel right up before any head movement occurs. Only then will the child's head tilt back.

We limit the freedom of our necks – and so of all of our body – when we treat our eyes as though they are passive, unfocused passengers in our heads.

Notice, by the way, how much more peripheral vision you have when you remember to release and lengthen your neck and think of that string taking you up from the crown of your head, as described in Chapter 3.

REORGANISE YOUR LIFE
Think ahead to the next working day and prepare
to focus and engage in your surroundings before
you get there and get caught up in your habitual
ways. Keep the novelty going by rewording your
Post-it, e.g. Sharpen up! Eyes right!

CHAPTER 9
GETTING ABOUT

THE PROBLEM
You may not think you have a problem with walking. Most of us say we feel better when moving about; it's when we're sitting that we suffer. But the way we're using our limbs when getting about often promotes tension in the spine and we then carry this stress pattern into other activities such as sitting. The reverse is also true, of course – sitting habits carry through to affect walking; it's just that moving about feels a more positive, happier activity. (For a more in-depth analysis of stress-free sitting, see Chapter 5.)

THE EXERCISES
Exercise 1:
Find a level, comfortable surface (a carpeted floor is ideal). You may prefer to remove your shoes. Stand with your hands by your sides, feet a few centimetres apart (not wide apart, but not uncomfortably close together). Distribute your

weight equally between your two feet and be aware of the balance of your head on your neck, avoiding any tendency to lean into your dominant side. Take a moment to ensure that your knees feel relaxed – that is, not locked back or pulled in towards each other.

Allow your spine to lengthen, be aware of the balance of your head and allow your tailbone to drop. Let your hands drop to your sides with your thumbs pointing forwards.

Particularly notice where the weight of your body is referred down through your feet. If you are standing in a poised and balanced way, the weight is predominantly down through your heels and not the balls of your feet. It is distributed in a ratio of around 60 per cent through the heels and 40 per cent through the rest of your feet (excluding the arch). This may seem unfamiliar – you may feel as though you are falling backwards; this is most likely to be because you are used to putting too much weight onto your toes.

Notice if your pelvis is twisted. To check this, put your hands on the brim of your pelvis (what you may have once called your hips) to monitor if one is more forward than the other.

If this is the case, you are standing with a twist. Ease back on the side that was twisted forward until your torso is straightened.

Spread your hands and place the palms on the small of your back and ease *back* into them. As you release middle back tension you will find that your ribs drop down in front.

Let your arms drop by your sides again, thumbs forward. Now you are standing comfortably, we can begin.

You are going to monitor the movements you make as you practise some exaggerated walking on the spot. Apart from keeping your head balanced and back long, do not worry too much about exactly how you walk on the spot. Take it slowly and bring your knees higher than you do when walking normally.

Notice two things:
– Whether there is any forward lurch of your spine with each leg lift; there should be gentle muscle movement and lengthening, but no lurching.
– How much your knees tense in towards each other at the start of each leg lift. They should not pull in at all.

Once you are happy that you've achieved these two objectives, it is time to move on to the next exercise.

Exercise 2:
Once again, begin by standing as before, poised and balanced, hands by your sides. Think about taking a step but don't move yet. When you do move it will be very slowly.

Without moving your torso forwards at all, shift your weight slightly onto your right foot and place your left foot on the ground in front of you. If your chin, neck or torso has leaned forwards to accomplish this – or worse still, all three – start again. Your foot starts the movement, not your chin or pelvis.

Your body weight stays back on your right foot. Lift the heel of your right foot and as you do so, feel your body being lifted and moved forward so that the weight comes to rest on your left foot. Your right foot is impelling you forward in a smooth, rocking movement. Feel your right foot being pleasantly worked as it lifts and rolls you up, forward and down.

Now your weight is entirely on your left foot. Move forward again by placing your right foot in front of your left, lift your left heel and transfer the weight to your right foot. Remember to only allow your torso forwards *with* the movement, not ahead of it.

Now you are off and walking very slowly but with poise. It may feel odd but this is a slow-motion version of good walking. When you feel comfortable with this, gradually increase your pace to your normal walking speed.

Exercise 3.
This is an observational exercise which helps to clarify some of the principles in Exercise 2.

Find a clear, safe space in which to walk backwards. Begin by standing as before, hands by sides, looking straight ahead. Walk backwards at whatever pace makes you feel secure and comfortable. Then decide to walk forwards, changing direction in as smooth and uninterrupted a fashion as possible. As you walk forwards, take with you the positive feelings that walking backwards promoted; weight more back on your heels, a finer sense of balance (especially with regard to your head balanced on your spine – your head, neck and spine operating as one unit).

Two things to notice:
– You will see your feet moving on the lower edge of your peripheral vision as you walk forwards in a way that you can't if your chin and chest are being thrust out ahead of your feet. Seeing your feet in this way is a good indicator that your walking is becoming less of an effort and less thrusting –

the precise opposite of the appalling chin up and chest out approach.

– Secondly, be conscious of where the weight of your body is coming down through your feet. When you move in a more tension-free manner, you will feel more of the outside of your feet as you walk.

Exercise 4:

Stand as before and place your right foot in front of you. Transfer your weight evenly between your feet by bending your right knee slightly. The left leg stays straight. The weight in each foot is predominantly down through the heels.

Your torso is balanced between your two feet and your body is facing forwards, not twisted at all.

Start to move your right knee and lower leg in a slow, thoughtful, clockwise circle, pivoting around your ankle, exploring the full mobility of your joints.

You should be able to do this without lifting your right big toe on the farthest reach of the circle.

If your toe is lifting off the ground on the outward rotation, stop and think what muscles you need to release in order to be able to accomplish it. Is there resistance in your knee, your lower back, or tension in your neck? Use the exercise as a way of exploring how your balanced body can be more flexible.

You may feel the muscles in the back of your left leg being stretched as your right knee approaches the twelve o'clock position.

Be aware of any tendency to press down on the arch of your left foot. If this is happening, your left knee is tending towards the centre line of your body. Keep it directed away.

Now take your right knee around again in an anticlockwise direction and explore how much movement is available on the inward rotation, without crushing down on the arch of your right foot. As you work, imagine you are on a beach and making a perfect footprint in the sand. Now bring your foot back and be amazed at how different it feels. In a very few minutes, working slowly with your mind engaged, a very simple exercise like this can be incredibly productive.

Now work the other foot in the same manner.

THE PRINCIPLE
Even in a sedentary job we may take thousands of steps a day and take them in a manner that is an effort and puts stress on the spine.

The first two exercises focus on a common mistake in walking: moving the spine towards the leg rather than vice versa. In poised, balanced walking, your spine is carried along effortlessly. Think of length coming out of your back and travelling along the underside of your thigh and your walking will feel buoyant and light.

The third exercise demonstrates how you can move without strain. In walking backwards you are doing something that you so rarely do, that you will not have had the chance to learn and incorporate any damaging habits. The experience of feeling your body move in an unfamiliar, habit-free way helps you to map these sensations onto your usual walking action.

Exercise 4 recognises how much we restrict the flexibility of our lower limbs, unconsciously limiting the lateral movement of our knees and tightening our ankles. This exercise offers a way of regaining that flexibility.

REORGANISE YOUR LIFE

Make friends with your feet – they are doing an important job so trust them more. You wouldn't spend all day wearing gloves, and yet we often spend most of our waking hours wearing shoes. Give your feet a break – go shoeless when you can. Five minutes padding about barefoot on a carpeted floor can do wonders for recharging your energy levels.

Vary your shoes as often as possible; keep a separate pair at the office and a different pair for driving. When buying shoes, think about giving your feet some breathing space. Your upright body balances through your feet; by allowing them to be as unconstricted as possible, your whole sense of balance will improve.

Incidentally, your legs are not meant to be stood upon. They are a delicate system of levers for moving us around the planet. The tonic quality of the muscles is lost if you use them as solid pillars for supporting your body when standing still. Keep moving over your ankles, if only very slightly – do not let your legs become fixed and locked.

Be careful carrying a bag over your shoulder; not only may you find that you are hitching your shoulder up, but if the bag is bulky you may be walking and standing in a twisted way to accommodate it. If so, reorganise by wearing it more centrally, to the front or back of your body or invest in a new bag.

*The things we wear and carry
are not supposed to damage us!*

CHAPTER 10
THE WORLD ON YOUR SHOULDERS

THE PROBLEM

Most of us go around much of the time with tense shoulders, usually without realising it.

As you become more tense, your shoulders creep closer to your ears, your neck tenses up and your shoulders and chest narrow, and this constricts how easily you breathe. Your shoulders are doing more work than they need to and you feel more tired as a consequence.

Shoulder tension is also a significant contributor to some forms of repetitive strain injury. And remember: tense shoulders not only make you feel bad, they make you look bad; less confident and less assertive. The secret isn't to walk around in an appalling parade-like posture, but to find a way to relax the shoulders and stop them wasting so much of your energy.

THE EXERCISES

Exercise 1:

A really easy exercise to begin.

Sitting, place your hands on your knees, palms down. Slowly rotate your hands outwards until they are resting palms upwards. Notice how this widens you across the top of the chest.

Now stand. As your arms drop by your sides, allow your hands to rotate outwards slightly until your thumbs are forwards.

Exercise 2:
You can do this next exercise sitting or standing, although you may find standing easier until you've practised.

Stand with your feet slightly apart, weight evenly on both feet, hands by sides, thumbs forward and head balanced on lengthening neck. Gradually bring your left shoulder and left ear together at the same time. Make sure your other shoulder doesn't move in the meantime.

With your head still on one side, let your left arm and shoulder drop down the side of your body as far as you can.

Notice how far down the length of your body your hand has been allowed to drop. Leaving your arm and shoulder in their new, relaxed length, only now restore your head to the upright position.

Continue the exercise with the right side. Be aware that this time your left shoulder might want to get in on the act. As you do this, you may feel your shoulders and neck being stretched. This is good. We're so familiar with the feeling of shoulders being high we don't notice it, so this exercise is a habit-breaker.

Repeat the exercise at regular intervals and as you feel you need it. Start earlier in the day and catch yourself before you start the old familiar tension-filled routine.

Exercise 3:

For this splendid exercise you will need to be brave and ignore the derision of your colleagues. Ideally, enlist a friend to observe you.

Stand up with your arms dropping by your sides, hands relaxed. Rotate your hands so that your thumbs point forwards and you feel your elbows rotating further into your sides. Relax your shoulders and allow your arms to be their true length (as in Exercise 2). Move your right arm very slowly sideways, away from your body, stopping the minute you (or your friend) observe that your right shoulder is rising.

Allow the underside of your arm to lengthen as though a friendly puppeteer is taking your arm out through strings on the fingertips.

Let your arm come out at right angles to your body (it may tend to move forwards but think of it drifting back into place).

This is very gentle, but what you are doing is radically changing the way you use your body. You're using your shoulder as a lever, not a hoist. You can expect to feel quite a pull and maybe some discomfort at first, particularly on the underused underside of your arm. Now continue the exercise by working with the other arm.

This exercise can be extended in the following way:

Take your hand outwards until it is around 30 cm from your body. Then rotate your hand at the wrist until the palm is facing forwards. Let your shoulder drop and, with your hand still facing forwards, bring your arm behind your back, as though you are about to pat yourself just below your bottom. (If you are patting yourself on the bottom, your shoulder and arm are not relaxed enough.)

Rotate your hand again at the wrist, so the back of your hand is against your body. Hinge at the elbow and start to move your hand and forearm up your back, as though feeling for a zip. Move as far as you can and then relax and drop your elbow and shoulder. This will, in the short term, move your arm further down your back. However, if you

proceed in this way, constantly relaxing and dropping your elbow and shoulder and then moving up again you will find that you will actually, ultimately, reach much higher than you were previously able to in the old, go-for-it way.

Now continue this exercise with the other arm.

As you get used to the feel of these exercises, you'll learn to involve your shoulders less in everyday movements. You'll relax more across the top of your arms and shoulders and your arms will regain their natural length.

THE PRINCIPLE

Most of the activities we perform are performed over and over again in the same situation – at a desk, at a drawing board, at the kitchen sink. We allow ourselves to become drawn into whatever it is that we are working on. Our shoulders become rounded, our chests narrow – we can be a good two shirt or blouse sizes narrower than we need be – and our shoulders creep higher. Not only are your shoulders up around your ears but the whole of the upper torso is narrower because your chest and back muscles are all contracting in towards the centre. After a while this misuse becomes familiar and habitual.

What's more, we don't look good. Because we have narrowed our upper torso, we look less assertive. When the shoulders are hunched, the pectoral or chest muscles are shortened, which makes the whole of the torso looks narrower. When we are tense and the muscles are contracted – the effect is as though a fan has closed. When the shoulder and chest muscles release, they lengthen and you look wider across the top of your chest and shoulders. The fan has opened into its natural state.

These exercises help us to unlearn shoulder tension. Moving the arms sideways, as in Exercise 3, gets us used to the idea of lengthening the muscles on the underside of our arms instead of using our shoulders to lift our hands. This is particularly important when sitting at a desk, lifting the hands to begin to type, write or draw; the unhelpful habit of tightening hands, wrists and arms establishes just the right muscular environment to encourage repetitive strain injury!

Releasing and dropping your shoulder and elbow when performing arm actions may seem counter-intuitive, but you reach much farther by doing so and you are maintaining your arm's true length and the tonic quality of your muscles. You are also able to perform actions which you might have previously given up on, just because you were performing them in a tight, impatient and tense way. For more on this, see Chapter 7.

POSTURE POST IT

widen across
the top
of the arms

REORGANISE YOUR LIFE

Make your office environment feel yours —
anything which gives you your own space and
makes you feel you're in control of your own
territory; screens, plants, shelves, even
photographs. This will help you feel more open,
positive and relaxed.

Before you do any work at a desk, stop and
think of relaxing those shoulders and lengthening
the underside of your arm. Concert pianists can

sit for a long period before raising their hands to the keyboard. Part of this is to reorganise the body to perform. Think particularly of letting weight drop into the points of your elbows before moving your hands on top of the keyboard, and let your arms hinge easily at the elbow without any pulling up to the shoulder.

Most office activities can be used as an excuse to work on yourself, ridding yourself of damaging habits. When using the telephone, for example, bring the phone to your ear the long way round: be aware of the balance of your head on the top of your neck, shoulders relaxed. And remember, when carrying anything, make sure the weight is equally balanced – and that includes your arms.

CHAPTER 11
FLEXIBLE FRIENDS

THE PROBLEM
Not feeling so mobile these days? Stiffness, aches and pains in the joints can, in extreme cases, signal the onset of repetitive strain injury.

THE EXERCISES
Exercise 1:
Standing or sitting, think of your spine lengthening and shoulders and elbows dropping as you hold your hands in front of you, arms bent at the elbow. Begin with palms facing each other.

FLEXIBLE FRIENDS

Pretend that you have got water on your hands and shake them from side to side to dry them, keeping your wrists relaxed. Don't shake too hard – use the weight of your hands to explore the limits of movement you have in your wrists. Keep the palms facing each other throughout this exercise.

Then turn your hands palm downwards and shake them again, this time in a vertical direction.

Then repeat the first movement, with palms facing.

Exercise 2:

Sitting or standing as before, hold your hands in front of you, palms facing each other. Imagine you have a large, lightweight beach ball between your hands (the beach ball's diameter is the same as the width across your chest).

Keeping your hands the same distance apart, start to move them as though you are rotating the beach ball, first rotating about one axis, then another – as if the ball's surface is covered in writing and you are examining every word.

This will take your elbows, wrists and the ball and socket joint of your arms into some previously unvisited places!

Keep the three-dimensional image of the ball strong in your mind so that your palms stay the same distance apart.

Exercise 3:
Standing, bring one hand up in front of you, palm facing away from you.

Imagine standing in front of a shop window. Your hand is going to wipe along the width of it.

Start to move your hand along the glass, away from

the centre of your body.
Keep the image strong – the
palm of your hand is going
to continue along the glass,
as if you are cleaning it with
a smooth cloth.

Do not allow your shoulder
to rise as your hand moves
away from you. When you
feel you are approaching the limit of your
movement, relax (and drop) your shoulder to
allow more length in the underside of your upper
arm, which in turn allows your hand to extend a
few centimetres farther.

Don't expect to be able to reach too much farther, especially on the first attempt. It is the final part of the exercise which is important and you will find you can extend your hand a little farther each time. The length is achieved by dropping your shoulder and not by leaning outwards.

THE PRINCIPLE
Performing the opposite move to the one you keep repeating all the time promotes mobility and extends underused muscles. Over time, when you are performing repetitive actions day after day, a limited set of muscles may be used. The mobility of your joints can become restricted, resulting in stiffness and pain. The immobility comes from overusing one set of muscles and underusing others.

Bringing your awareness into these areas and exploring their natural range of movement helps keep them flexible. To do this, you need to take the movement to its limit (not below it) in a carefully monitored fashion. Do not overdo it.

REORGANISE YOUR LIFE

Ask yourself where your joints have not moved to today. Look at how you perform repetitive actions. What are the opposite actions? Can you identify the underused muscles? If so, give them a brief workout and give those overused muscles a holiday.

As well as the exercises above, find time to explore one joint per day. For example, Wednesday is elbow day. Really get to know how flexible this marvel of natural engineering can be. Release the muscles and remember to allow your spine, shoulder and arms to lengthen as you move and explore your joints.

CHAPTER 12
LIFT OFF

THE PROBLEM

Lifting anything – whether heavy or not – is a health and safety issue. You may already have suffered the consequences of lifting inappropriately; backache, muscle spasms, a slipped disc. In this chapter we will look at lifting objects, including the way that you do so when the only object you have to lift is yourself.

THE EXERCISES

Exercise 1:

This exercise will help you learn to bend and straighten without tightening your lower back.

Find a clear wall and stand with your feet 5 to 8 cm from it. Lean back so that the wall supports you. Your feet should be hip-width apart, hands dropping by your sides, head balanced and neck lengthening (but both head and neck clear of the wall).

Lower yourself down the wall into a shallow squat – you will not be descending very far, perhaps 10 cm at most. Think of your knees gently buckling to allow you to slide down the wall. Do not force anything. The weight of your body should be mainly down through your heels.

If you find your back is losing contact with the wall, it is because you are tensing your lower back and arching your spine. If this happens, halt your descent, release the tension and lean back into the wall before continuing.

Come to a halt and, as slowly as possible, reverse the move. The weight of your body should again be in your heels. Be aware of your contact with the wall. You are using the wall as a reference point to check if your lower back is tensing as you bring yourself back into a fully standing position. Especially at the last moment – as you are about to stand fully – use the wall to help you resist the temptation to tighten and arch away from the wall. Keep your back in contact with the wall. This may cause your legs to tremble slightly but as you get used to standing without tensing, the trembling will cease.

Exercise 2:
Find a flight of stairs where you can work on this exercise undisturbed. Stand at the foot of the stairs. Think of a string taking the crown of your head upwards.

Feel the weight of your body principally through your heels. Shift your weight slightly to transfer it onto your left leg. Keeping your head balanced, neck and back aligned, and without any forward lurch of your spine, bring your right foot up and place it on the first step.

This is the critical point – the start of the action. If your right knee pulls inwards as you bring your foot up, this is an indication of unnecessary tension and effort. In which case, repeat the action, thinking of releasing the tension in your upper leg as you lift your foot.

(Practising this action until you can lift your foot without tensing your knee inwards is beneficial in

itself. It is a habit-breaker.)

Place your foot – the whole length of your foot, not just the ball of your foot – onto the stair. Take a step upwards with the weight of your body going down principally through your right heel. (If the tread of the stairway is too narrow to allow this, find another staircase.)

Continue up the staircase being conscious of:
– the imaginary string taking you upwards from the crown of your head
– weight going down through your heels
– your knees drifting outwards from the centre line of your body.

Coming down again:
Avoid the mistake of thrusting your head and neck forwards in order to look at the stairs. Instead, hinge forwards slightly from the hips.

Toes and then heel contact each step as you lower yourself downstairs. Keep in mind that your weight goes mainly down through your heels and keep thinking up (remember the imaginary string on the crown of your head). Don't forget those knees drifting away from each other.

Progress seems slow at first but your posture is very secure and you will be doing far less work as a result.

Exercise 3:

Take two books and place one of them on the floor. Place the other on the seat of a chair so that it is just below your reach. Approach the book on the floor and stand as close as possible – we usually stand too far away from the object we are going to pick up.

Place your feet farther apart – you will almost certainly have instinctively stood with your feet too close together. You don't have to square up to the book, the most important factor is the distance between your heels.

Think of the imaginary string from the crown of your head keeping your head balanced and neck long, then begin to go into a squat. Make sure that you keep your feet fully in contact with the floor, the weight of your body dropping down through your heels and not transferring too much onto your toes. If, as you squat, your heels come off the ground, your feet are probably too close together. Move them farther apart and start again. If you are wearing shoes with pronounced heels, take them off.

As you descend, your body pivots slightly at the hips to allow you to reach forwards between your knees and pick up the book. Your weight always remains principally down through your heels and the weight of your back falls behind the line of your hips.

BUSY BODY

Pick up the book and reverse the action to stand up: think of the string on the crown of your head taking you up, and your weight moving down through your heels and not forward onto your toes. As you straighten your legs, think of your tailbone dropping, as you practised in Exercise 1. Your head, neck and back stay relaxed and lengthening throughout.

Now for the second book. In many ways this is trickier because of our preconceptions; it requires you to make a revised visual judgement as to how you perform the action.

Once you have gauged that the book is out of reach – however marginally – perform a mini-squat to lower your body and enable yourself to pick up the book. This way, you are using your legs to do the work and keeping your spine free from unnecessary tension. It avoids the maladroit regime of a jutting-out chin, bending from the waist and legs held stiffly to keep you balanced, which is potentially damaging and looks ungainly.

THE PRINCIPLE

Heels down, knees away from each other.

If you have been following the chapters of this book in sequence, you will find these ideas familiar by now. When you are lifting anything, including your own body, your legs do the work. If you

140

become unbalanced through your weight being too far forward onto your toes, your lower back is likely to go into spasm to protect itself as it is made to perform an action that is potentially damaging.

When standing up, tightening the lower back is such a compulsive habit that most of us are not even aware when we are doing it. Exercise 1 helps us to become aware of what we are doing to ourselves and to relearn an apparently simple action. We are also reminding ourselves that lifting does not just involve other objects – it also means ourselves. See Chapter 6 for more on this.

In Exercise 2, we find that if we are trying to lift ourselves through our toes, our legs are bound to tighten. The result is that our back will also be tense. There is no need for this – the action can be undertaken in a much less stressful and less energy-wasting fashion. The exercise also demonstrates that poised movements feel more secure. We could stop at any moment in this exercise without feeling off-balance.

Exercise 3 encourages you to use that funny pair of hinges halfway up your legs. Use those knees! It also highlights the danger that the nearer the object, the more likely you are to take potentially damaging short cuts. This applies to any activity which involves losing height. Squatting into such tasks is not only ergonomically appropriate, it also keeps your hips mobile. Many people become stiff in their hips partly because they keep their legs tense instead of using their knees when bending.

REORGANISE YOUR LIFE

Most of us have evolved complicated sets of habits around everyday activities. Bending and straightening actions are probably the most revealing of these habits. People do not use their knees enough! Keep this in mind when approaching even apparently innocuous activities such as writing a cheque at a supermarket checkout – how many of them have a writing surface at a level which does not involve you having to lower your own height? It may seem strange at first but it is more natural and graceful to do a semi squat rather than a bend from the waist.

Every change of height is an opportunity to practise keeping yourself flexible.

CHAPTER 13
DON'T HOLD YOUR BREATH

THE PROBLEM
Breathlessness, fatigue, feeling of remoteness, light-headedness, poor circulation?

These can all be caused by bad breathing habits.

When we conduct workshops, the two ideas people most readily relate to are sitting badly and not breathing properly.

THE EXERCISE
You can work on this exercise either sitting or lying down. Lying in a semi-supine position (see Chapter 4) is ideal because your ribs are potentially at their most relaxed in this position.

Start by thinking of widening and lengthening your body. Become aware of your breathing; don't be judgemental about it, you're observing, not getting self-critical. Do not try to alter anything, although you may find your breathing changes for the better simply due to this self-monitoring. Focus more on the out than the in breath, as though exhaling is full of subtlety and interest. Notice how it varies from one breath to another – the length of each one, for example. This may cause your breath to naturally slow down. Do not forget the pause at the end of each exhalation before letting the breath back in, to avoid hyperventilation.

After a few minutes of observation, begin enhancing the out breath by adding a whispered sound, the sound 'ahh'. Let the sound escape through slightly parted lips, almost like a sigh – you are letting go of the breath, not forcing it out; think of the contrast between letting air out of a balloon and the effort of blowing it up.

Think of your out breath as having length; imagine your breath moving along the whole length of your spine.

After half a dozen whispered 'ahh' sounds, turn your attention to your in breath. It will already be more natural and efficient as a result of your more complete out breath, but enhance it further by noticing your ribs (the complete span, including the ribs in your back and sides) moving out towards your elbows, like sails

caught in the wind. Again, you are allowing this to happen and not forcing anything.

Imagine your in breath as having width, travelling easily through the breadth of your body.

Out is long, in is wide. Let go on the out breath, clearing the lungs of old air, leaving room for reviving air on the in breath. Think of letting go of stressful, negative thoughts as you let the breath go out – let them float away on the whispered 'ahh'.

THE PRINCIPLE

We under-breathe in times of stress and develop bad breathing habits. For example, when we concentrate we tend to hold our breath. We under-breathe when people invade our space. Paradoxically, smokers often under-breathe when not smoking because they have started to rely on the exhalation of cigarette smoke in order to fully exhale. When smokers give up, they often find it hard to get back to natural breathing.

It is not useful to 'take a deep breath' – that just promotes more tension. 'Chin up, chest out, take a deep breath' is the very reverse of natural breathing.

The 'ahh' sound raises the soft palate (the softer part of your upper mouth) and helps free the airways. This breathing practice is not something you do all the time but it helps retrain your body to breathe more fully and naturally, working against the ingrained habit of under-breathing. It stimulates your body to better everyday use.

POSTURE POST IT

let go with the out breath

REORGANISE YOUR LIFE

Smell your environment. Are you not breathing fully because you don't want to? Bad air days need strategy; nice smells (oils, plants, flowers), ionisers, or reminders of better atmospheres (photographs of seaside or countryside).

If you do find that you are in a situation where your space is invaded (crushed on the tube or in a lift) and you feel deprived of oxygen, don't hold your breath or take shallow breaths; focus on breathing more completely and make the best of every out breath to rid yourself of inhaled toxins and stale air.

CHAPTER 14
WHERE NEXT?

You never stop. As we said in the introduction, you keep working on yourself. You have learnt damaging postural habits by repetition and repetition is the only way you will unlearn them. Repeat the exercises and continue to think about the way you move and perform everyday tasks. You never reach the end of the journey; there is always something new to learn, a new challenge to meet and a new situation to react to.

And you need never be bored again. Whilst standing at a bus stop, sitting in a plane, enduring the world wide wait at the computer, think of your back, your head, your neck, the manner in which you are sitting or standing, the way of performing an action with the least tension and stress. Observe yourself as you are about to fall into old habits and enjoy the process of doing things in new ways.

The exercises and ideas in *The Busy Body* are predominantly derived from direct experience of the Alexander Technique. Remarkable, empowering and life-enhancing though this book certainly is (we're sure you'll agree), it can only scratch the surface. You will gain even more and travel so much farther with the aid of an accomplished teacher. The Technique is a collaborative process and you will find the skills and insight of a good teacher absolutely invaluable.

You can find your nearest teacher of the Technique by contacting STAT, the professional association:

The Society of Teachers of the Alexander Technique
Tel: 020 7284 3338
www.stat.org.uk

The inspiration for much of this book has arisen from working with colleagues, friends and pupils. This too is an ongoing process and you can keep up with our latest ideas on our website at:

www.thebusybody.co.uk

APPENDIX 1
BODY MAP

PECTORAL
MUSCLES

BICEPS

NICE LITTLE
MUSCLE
(see Chapter 1)

BRIM
OF
PELVIS

HIPS

THE BUSY BODY

CROWN
OF HEAD

ATLANTO-
OCCIPITAL
JOINT

NECK
VERTEBRAE

BACK
VERTEBRAE

LUMBAR
VERTEBRAE

SACRUM

COCCYX

RIB
CAGE

CROWN
OF HEAD

OCCIPUT

BACK
OF NECK

JAW
JOINT

BRIM OF
PELVIS

HIP

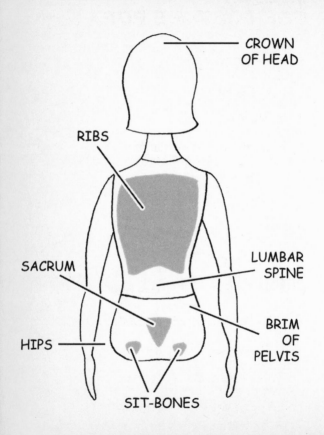

APPENDIX 2
THE POSTURE POST-ITS

1   Watch yourself

2   Stop and think

3   Think up

4   Lie down and recharge

5   Use those sit bones

6   Pivot at the hips

7   Relax and go further

8   Eyes lead

9   Move forward but stay back

10 Widen across the top of the arms

11 Explore all the parts

12 Use those knees

13 Let go with the out breath

ACKNOWLEDGEMENTS

For sharing ideas and giving inspiration which directly led to this book, we would like to thank: Don Burton, Wendy Bonington, Joan Diamond and Michael Hardwicke Thanks to pupils, students on courses and all those at Cumbria Alexander Training who have, over the years, provided the catalyst for constantly developing the work. There are debts of other kinds to people in and out of organisations who have encouraged the Alexander work in general and The Busy Body in particular. For their encouragement and valuable feedback, we thank: Edna Burnett, Ann Clark, Martin Condit, Gillian Cowburn, Martin and Jane Dix, Joyce Harris, Peter Leney, Judith Maddison, Kate Morpeth, Michael Mumford, Kathleen Purdy, Carolyn Stone and Helen Vaughan. And finally thanks to John Benson and Pam Grant for putting up with us when we don't do as we say.